I0065556

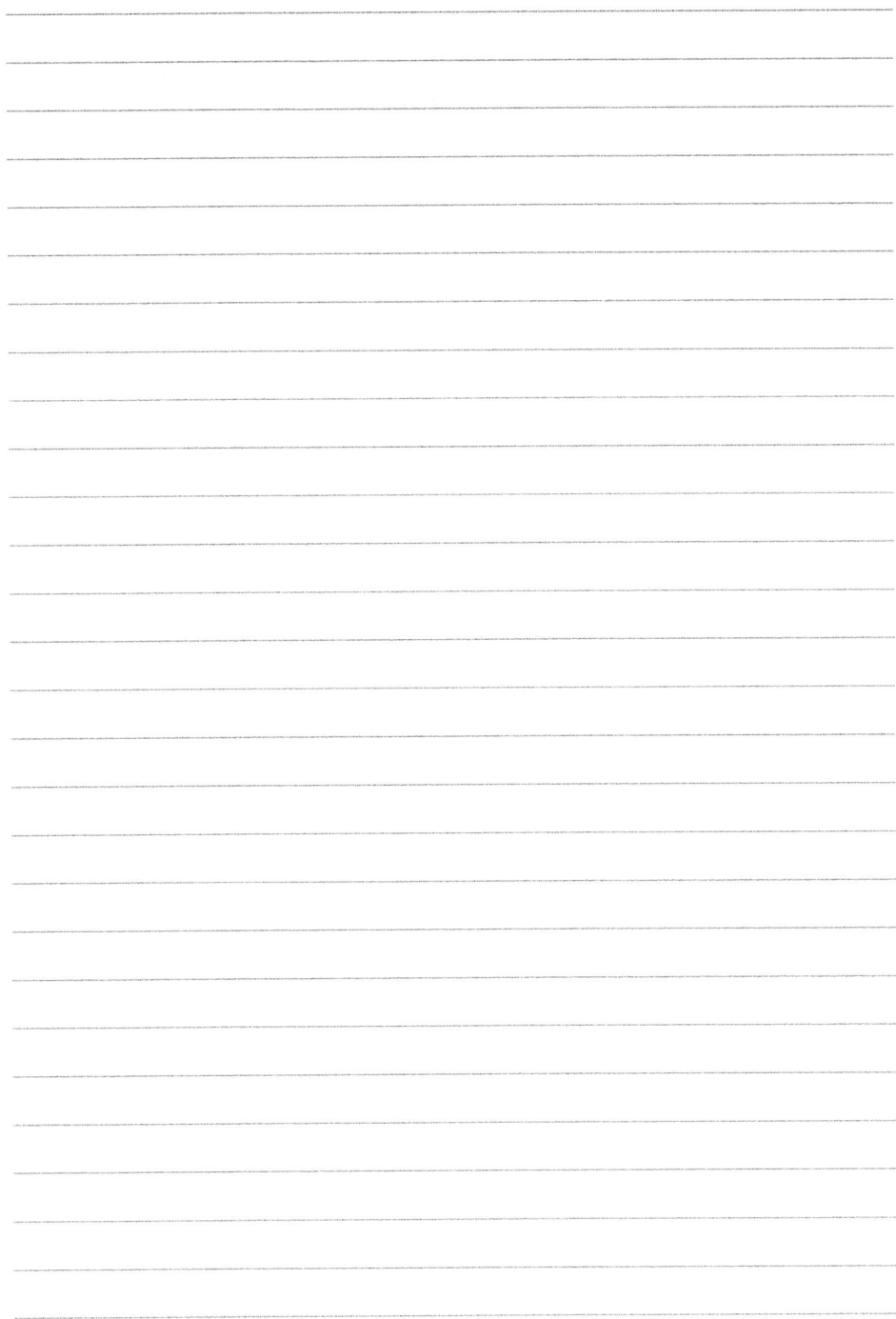

First Responder Doctor Journal Notebook
We Put Our Patients First: First Responder Journal Series
Gift Book Ideas For Doctors
Paperback ISBN: 978-1-989733-44-8
Copyright Dunhill Clare Publishing 2020
All Rights Reserved. Cover Design by Sharon Purtill